KIDS WON'T EAT HEALTHY?
Quick, Read This Book!

THE STRESSED-OUT PARENT'S GUIDE
TO DRAMA-FREE MEALS

BY Theresa Bonner
ILLUSTRATED BY Alissa Mendenhall

Copyright © Theresa Bonner, 2015
Edited by Carina Gonzalez and Rebekah Harrison
Illustrated by Alissa Mendenhall
All rights reserved

ISBN-13: 978-1517258443
ISBN-10: 1517258448

First Edition:
Library of Congress Cataloging-in-Publication Data

Bonner, Theresa
Kids Won't Eat Healthy? Quick, Read This Book! / Theresa Bonner–1st ed

Thanks mom and dad
for giving me your absolute best.

TABLE OF CONTENTS

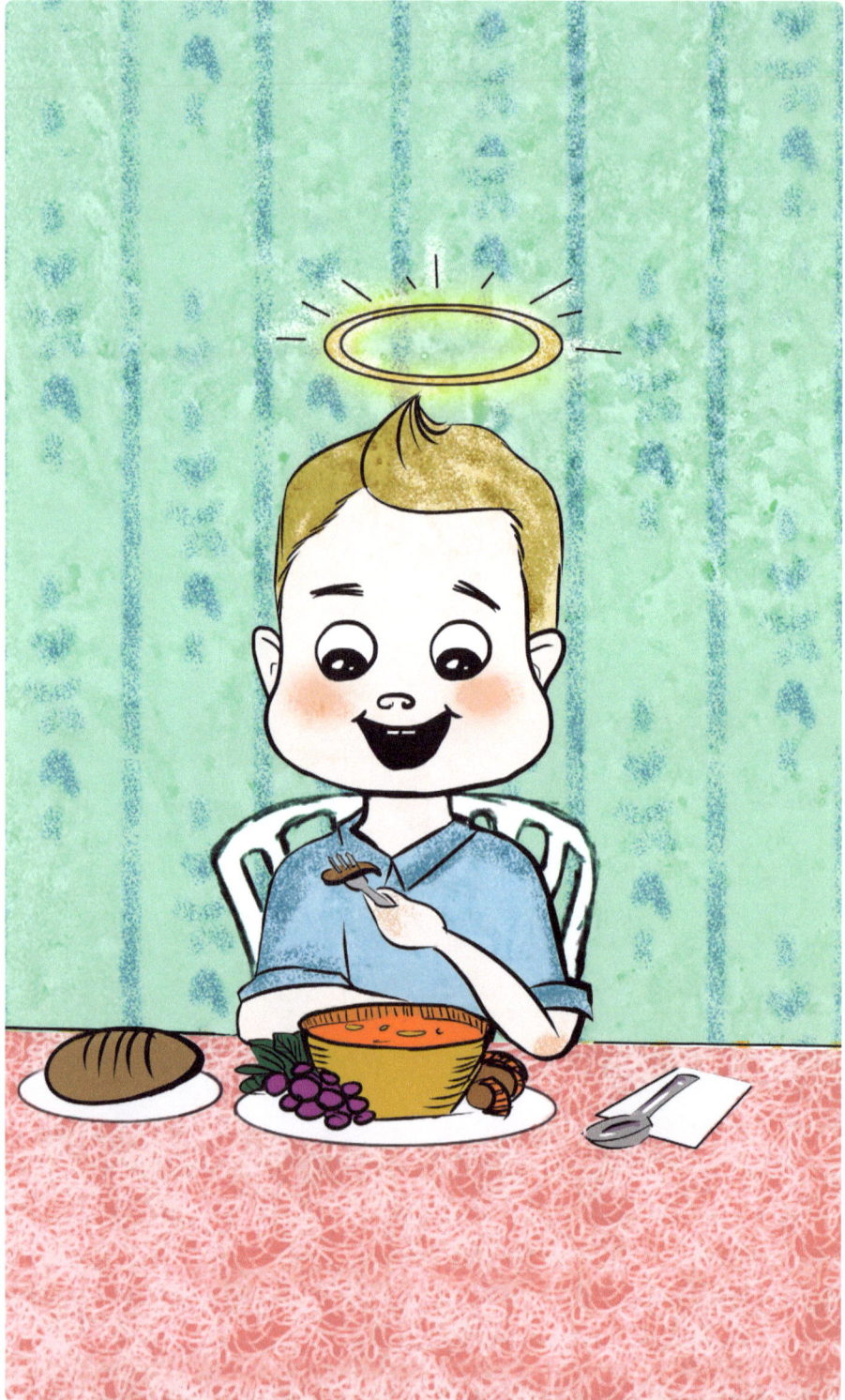

INTRODUCTION

One of the biggest struggles that most of us face as parents is getting our kids to sit down at the table and actually eat what we put in front of them. We want them to eat this well-thought-out, nutritious food that we took time and energy to make. Furthermore, we want them to smile sweetly (like the angels that they are) and thank us for our love and hard work. In this same glorious daydream, we live in a palacial estate on the beach with a gardener and a personal chef to bring said nutritious meals to the table; the one in the formal dining room with the fireplace and large but tasteful wine collection.

This is a lovely fantasy world to visit from time to time, but then reality takes over and we are back at our non-formal dining room table. It has piles of school papers on one side, a severely disheveled center piece, and just enough room for dinner plates and maybe a drinking glass for each person. At this table the beautiful child in front of you will try to bargain, cry, beg, lie and do almost anything to not have to eat part or all of the meal you just spent 20 minutes to an hour making for them. We're just trying to keep them healthy; to keep them from having too many absences from school. Mostly, we're desperate to keep them from becoming another statistic and maybe even have better health than we have ourselves.

There's nothing wrong with us wanting to do right by our kids in the hope that they will be strong, healthy, and intelligent adults that know how to make the right food choices. It's our job. It's in our DNA to want our offspring to live long healthy lives to keep our species going strong. It's a lot of pressure to put on ourselves but it's hard to avoid.

Every night, it's another push and pull. Another night of feeling like you are a failure as a parent. Another night of just wanting to give up and order pizza or Chinese (Chinese is healthier right?) to end all of the fighting. You do your best to make the meals fun, colorful and exciting. Sometimes, you just give them what they want and sneak something on the plate you know they hate in the hope that they don't notice. That way they will at least eat something that's good for them! OK, now take a breath. We've all been there. If not every night, then more nights than we'd like to admit. It's OK. We're going to be OK.

There is a way to teach our children that food is indeed fun, interesting, exciting and has the potential to create an awesome future for them if they let it. This isn't something that happens overnight, especially with older kids. I'm not going to lie. Toddlers are way more open to the magic of food than teenagers, but it will happen if we can all work together. Knowledge is the key ingredient here. Learning how and why to make healthier choices as a whole family will make it easier for the individual to maintain those good habits in the long run.

The best part is, I know you can do this. I have known families that were in hopeless ruts of processed food and anguish-filled meal times. I'm not exaggerating when I say that they dreaded even thinking about dinner. A picky eater, and frustrated parents, is a terrible but very common combination. They all knew a fight was inevitable. With some outside guidance, they were able to work through it. Slowly, one day at a time, they were able to change the dining room from a torture chamber into a family room.

Here's a little secret about me. I'm kind of a tough love kind of mom. I believe in honesty and directness in everything I do. So, if you are ready and open to new ideas, I'd love to help you turn your family's collective tears into smiles all around. At the very least, you may find some new ideas to improve your own health. You've got nothing to lose and a healthier, happier family to gain.

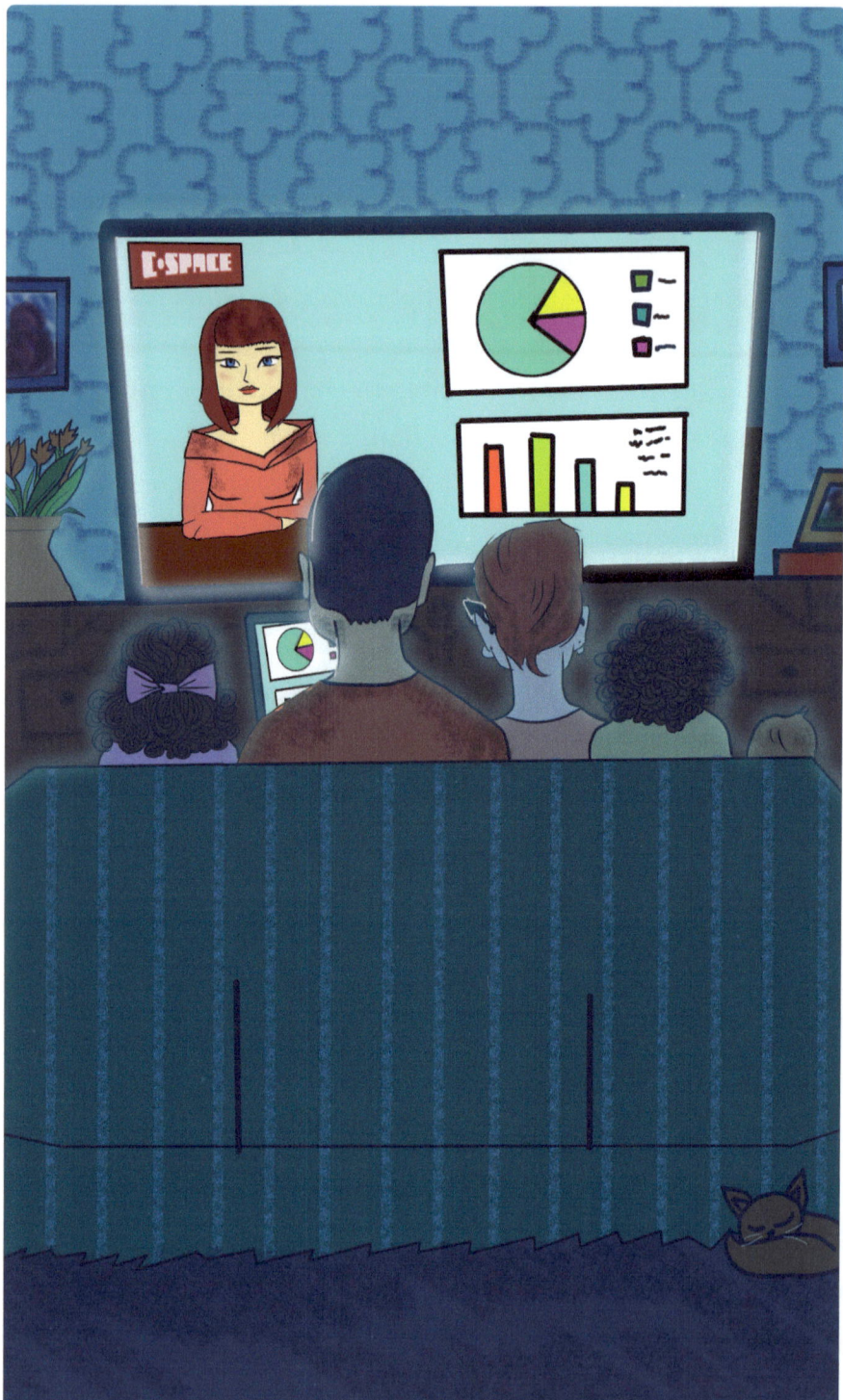

– Chapter 1 –
THE BAD NEWS FIRST

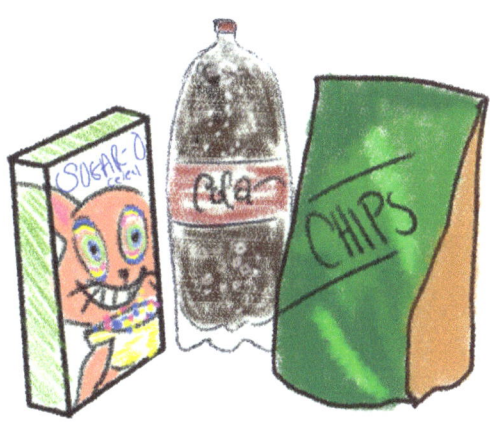

For the past decade, the media has been telling the American public that we are doomed. Doomed to become the most unhealthy country in the world; the fattest, sickest and most physically unfit group of people to ever live on this planet. It's been pretty harsh to hear that we have become so lackadaisical with our food choices and that we are destined to be "the first generation to outlive their own children" Harsh, but sadly true. Kids are getting sicker and heavier ever year.

Heart disease, diabetes, high cholesterol, high blood pressure and obesity in a 7-year-old would have been unheard of 3o years ago. Are children less active in general than they were back then? Simple answer; yes.

Though TV has been the main source of entertainment for kids since the 80's, now there is the internet that holds endless possibilities for distraction. It's on the computer, tablet, phone and the TV. They sit at school all day then come home and sit in front of screens of every size until they fall asleep at night. That makes a huge difference in the health of their little bodies. Somehow as a society, we've also given in to the fast food and processed food industries. In our own fatigue and stress, we've forgotten how (or decided we don't have time) to prepare a healthy meal. The statistics for childhood obesity can be truly terrifying if you are a parent or really just anyone who cares about the longevity of our children and this country.

Possibly even more alarming is the fact that America's incredibly poor eating habits are spreading all across the globe to countries that, until recently, had low rates of heart disease and cancer. So now our rampant inability to nourish ourselves is effecting the whole world. Countries that have always eaten mainly whole food diets, rich in healthy fats and nutrients are getting fatter and dying younger on the American diet. With every fast food hamburger meal or taco that is sold in Asia or Europe, the world gets one pound heavier. Just like America.

So, it's not just something that has happened to us. It's something that we are doing to ourselves. We have a choice every time we feel hunger or thirst to simply fill our stomaches or to nourish our bodies. As adults, we have far more control over what goes in to our bodies than children do. They rely on us to make sure they have the best food options to choose from. From the moment they are born, their health is in our hands. Understandably, money is a factor for far too many people. Sadly, it is more often the salty, sugary, artificially flavored and colored foods that are the cheapest. Many feel like this is the only food we can afford. It's hard to see that when we buy these over processed "foods" that we are actually paying for an empty box. There is nothing in there that our bodies want or can actually use to keep us alive. The sodas, energy drinks, just-add-water-and-heat meals, cheese puffs and pre-made lunch kits can be the biggest waste of money imaginable. They may cost less at the checkout, but in the long run they are insanely expensive.

When we eat these foods that are entirely devoid of nutrients, we need to eat more and more and more until we finally feel satiated. Low fat chips, or even vegetable puffs, are not health food! They are the food industries' way of luring us in with a bag that looks like it holds something good for us and then loading us up with gobs of salt, preservatives, and processed oils. The human body will never be satisfied by a handful of these snacks, because what it really wants is fat that it can assimilate, and some nutrients that will keep it going. So, we eat and eat and continue to eat until we feel either full or incredibly thirsty.

Then we pour ourselves a drink. Water would be the best option of course, but is that what most people reach for? Not usually. The majority of people would grab a soda, sweetened tea or a "juice" drink because many times when we take in a lot of salt we crave sweetness. So now we have a system full of sodium and more sugar than our bodies can process all at once. Insulin levels have spiked and blood pressure has risen. Maybe that wasn't the best afternoon snack. But now the bag is almost empty and we're nearly out of our favorite sugary drink. Time to go back to the store and buy some more! You see where I'm going with this?

By eating ourselves silly with processed foods devoid of any nutrients, we tend to end up in the doctor's office more often. How many times this year have you had to see the doctor for sinus infections, strep throat, digestive issues or even just complications from the common cold? How many days of school did your kids miss from the same issues? It is vital to have proper nutrition in order to stay healthy. Here's the truth. A healthy digestive track creates a healthy immune system. Without a healthy, well-rounded diet filled with real food, it is difficult to stay truly healthy. More doctor's visits means more doctor's bills and more prescriptions. Antibiotics, penicillin and steroids are not exactly cheap, are they?

What I am trying to get across to you is that I would much rather pay a bit more for good food than to pay hundreds (or thousands) of dollars a year for healthcare. I've actually always thought of my weekly grocery bill as preventative healthcare and that's what it is. My family and I rarely have the need to go to the doctor other than our yearly checkups. Yes, there is the occasional ear infection for my five-year-old (once every couple of years) but in general, we are healthier than most families I know. It is rare that we have to go to the drug store for an actual drug. This is something that I want for more people. For them to feel like they have control over their own health and the health of their family. They should feel that it's not just a roll of the dice to see if they will have a bright, vibrant future.

I know, not the way you wanted to start off a new book about getting your kids to eat better. I get it, I do. This first chapter has not been uplifting or positive. I need you to see and feel the seriousness of the situation, so that we can deal with it together in a serious way. Our family's health and well being should be one of our top priorities and in order for that to happen we need to have all of the facts. Call me crazy but I think that G.I. Joe had it right; "Knowing is half the battle." Pause for theme song to play in your head once or twice. Now that you know, what are you willing to do about it?

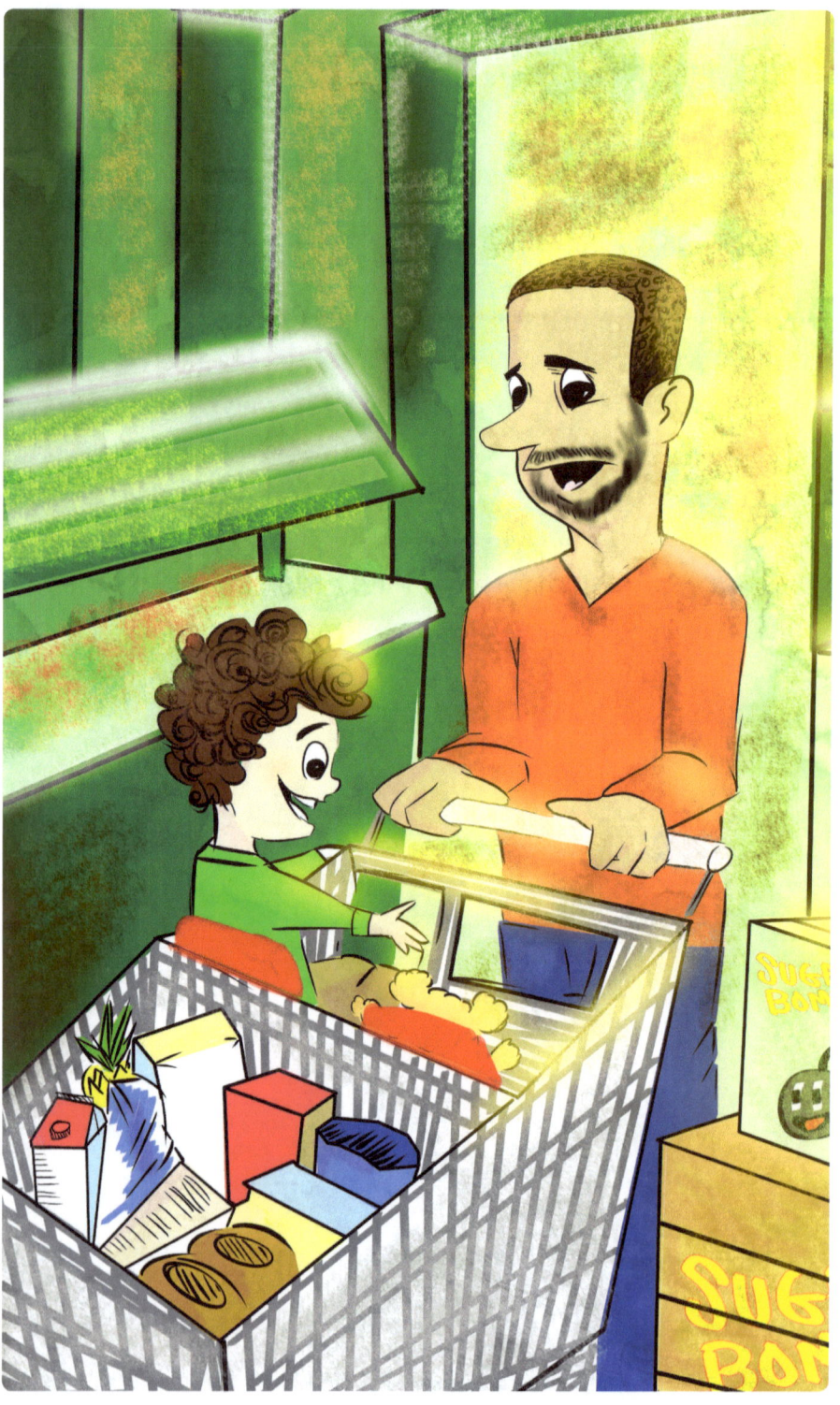

– Chapter 2 –
IMPROVING THE ODDS

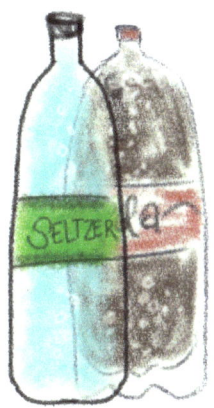

T rying to change your kid's eating habits all at once isn't going to work, much like an adult trying to go on a crash diet to lose 10 pounds before a wedding or bikini season isn't going to work. As soon as the wedding reception arrives, who do you think is going to be stationed at the buffet table guarding the cream puffs with their life? Who do you think will be gaining that ten pounds back, plus another five, in just a couple of weeks? If you try to take all of your kid's favorite things away all at once, they will fight and resent you. I'm talking exorcist kind of rage here. Let's try to make this shift as easy as we can on everyone.

Gradual changes are always the easiest to handle. If we take this one small step at a time, our families are going to be more willing to try new things more often, and sometimes not even realize that changes have happened. For instance, if your child is a juice-a-holic, start adding some water to their cup. This way you are decreasing the amount of sugar they are taking in gradually. Slowly keep adding more water as time goes on. If you take your time with it, they won't notice the change. Their taste will change along with their favorite juice. If they are soda drinkers, start making them homemade juice soda. This works with older kids too. It's very simple and if they are old enough, they will enjoy helping to make it with you. You simply combine seltzer water and juice. It couldn't be easier. It cuts the sugar intake by half and gets them in the habit of seeing it made. It takes away the ease of just grabbing a can or bottle out of the fridge. I'm not saying that your kids should be drinking lots of juice or carbonated beverages, but if it's something that is already part of their regular diet, it is easy to find ways of making their favorites healthier.

Another very good way of keeping the wrong choices out of your kid's hands and mouths is to stop buying them. I know, again with the tough love. If you have small children, the only way that they are going to have access to nutrient-poor foods is for you to bring them home and stock the cupboards with them. It's true that if your child is in school, they will have plenty of unhealthy options to choose from in the lunch room and at other people's homes. That's out of your control. What is well within your control is what you give your child. Again, I am not saying that you should go to your cupboard and throw out every single processed food item that you have and replace it with all organic, whole foods. I am saying that you can start to slowly, one box or bag at a time, stop buying them. You are in control of what you buy. You are the parent. You are the one making the money. You are the one responsible for your child's health.

Start out with something that is not a favorite, but something that the kids ask for occasionally. Oops, the store didn't have any of those today. Sorry! They don't have them the next time either. Am I endorsing lying to your children? Yeah, I guess I am. If you have the kind of child that can easily be reasoned with about the virtues of a naturally based, healthy diet, please go ahead and explain to them why you are no longer buying that treat. If you do, you probably don't need this book. For the rest of us, that interaction comes later.

This little exercise in removing the bad is as much for us as it is for them. For them, we are taking baby steps to having a diet filled with less sugar, sodium, preservatives and fillers. For us, it's a lesson in how we deserve to be in control of what we put in our shopping carts. Each time we subtract an unhealthy item from the pantry, they have one less poor food choice to make. At the same time, we are able to trust that we are doing our very best for our family. It isn't up to the media, society or the schools to keep our kids in top form. It's up to us, the parents. It would be wonderful if everyone was watching out for our kid's well being like we are but that's not even close to true. I think we all know that the people choosing what our kids are fed at school are not making the same choices that we would. Marketing executives do not have our sweet little cherub's best interest in mind when coming up with the latest slogan for [insert candy cereal here]. They are in it for the money. They don't care about our kids in the slightest. They see numbers and dollar signs where our kid's faces should be. The commercials, ads and store shelf placement, is all working against us. If we want our kids to avoid the traps that the food industry has in store for them, we have to start fighting for them. OK, still don't want to lie about why you didn't bring home that bag of X chips? That's cool. When they ask why you didn't buy it, say "because I love you." That's the truth, the whole truth and nothing but. At that moment, they might fight it and say just the opposite is true. In your heart, though, you'll know it's the absolute truth.

As long as we're being all honest here, I'm going to be straight with you. At this stage of the game there may be more tears than hugs and kisses coming from your beloved offspring, but we're not here for the snuggles. We're doing this to give them a fighting chance. We're here to learn and teach one of the most important lessons in life. How to keep ourselves healthy enough to live to be very, very old. That's something we all want, right? Not just to be old, but to be old and still kickin'! We want to be (and our kids to be) one of those amazing grandmas or grandpas that are running marathons in their 80's. Someone that hikes and gardens and goes dancing well into their 90's. We want to be on the news celebrating our 106th birthday. True, there's no way to guarantee any of these things will happen for us, but there are so many ways to improve our odds. It couldn't hurt to try, right?

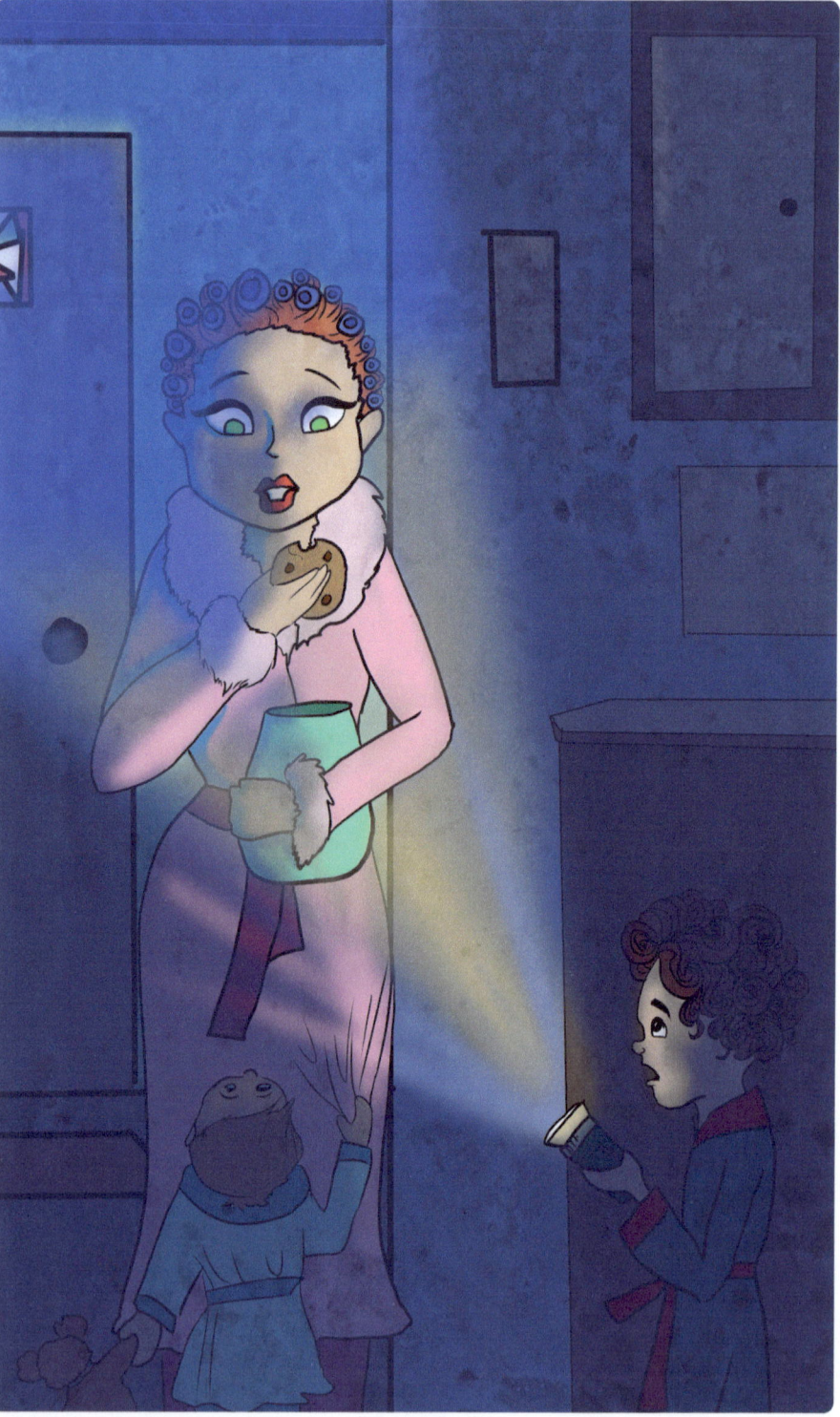

— Chapter 3 —
CHANGE STARTS WITH YOU

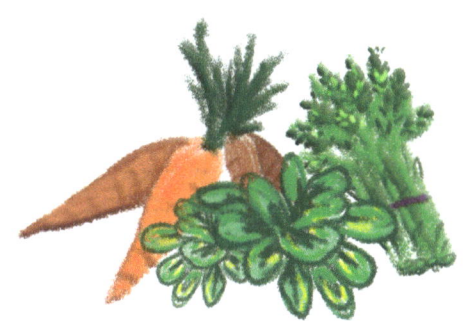

So you've started talking to your kids about healthy choices and that you are going to be buying less junk food for them. That's great! High five. Why then are you still sneaking off to get that extra value meal while they are at school? Is it going to mean as much to them that you are telling them, "no more sugary cereals" when you are eating a handful of chocolate chips while making their dinner? Are you a member of the "do as I say not as I do" club, or do you walk the talk? Our children look to us for the answers, big or small. They follow our example, sometimes way more than we'd like. You have a temper tantrum, they have a temper tantrum. You let a swear word slip, your ears are bleeding when they use that same expletive in passing. You eat a whole plate of pasta with not one bit of veggies or protein and they expect to be able to do the same thing. We are our children's heroes. If we are doing our job right, they want to be just like us when they grow up. No matter what we do, they probably will. If we overeat, chances are, so will they. If we say we hate fruits and vegetables, so will they. If we sit around watching TV or glued to the computer or phone... you get the picture.

Ask yourself, "What kind of role model do I want to be to my child?" Do you want them to look at you and be proud that you are strong, fast, smart, and love your body? If the answer is, "yes" then you need to put down this book for a minute and go find a mirror. Stand in front of that mirror and ask yourself, "Am I proud of the example that I'm setting for my kids?" If you can say, "yes" back at yourself then I applaud you. If the answer is, "eh..." then you know that you have some work to do on yourself before you can expect your kids to make the changes you want for them.

The first thing you need to do is to educate yourself. How can you teach them if you don't have the necessary information and skills? Would you want someone teaching your kids chemistry, that had no actual knowledge of science? Let me tell you, my high school chemistry teacher was actually the lacrosse coach. We had a great lacrosse team, but 85 percent of my class just scraped by because of a tremendous grading curve. I learned more about his ex-wife than I did about elements. I digress.

The first thing that you need to learn, is how the food you eat effects your body and mind. When you eat a whole plate of pasta with nothing else other than a big slice of garlic bread, how do you feel afterward? Are you full of energy? Can't wait to plan the next activity with your family? Do you feel light and fulfilled or do you just feel full? Are you lethargic and dragging around the kitchen, dreading the after-dinner dishes? What if you'd had a quarter of that portion of pasta on your plate with a big pile of fresh veggies and a little bit of protein? How do you think you might feel then? What if instead of pasta, you had some rice or quinoa? Do you experiment with different foods, or do you pretty much stick to the same old standard ingredients every week? Are you ready to open yourself up to more possibilities in the kitchen in order to see what foods make you feel your best? When was the last time that you can remember feeling really healthy? I mean REALLY healthy. No indigestion, heartburn, headaches, gas, bloating, fogginess, colds, sinus infections, anxiety, high blood pressure... I'll wait while you check your calendar. Sure, we all have times when we are feeling a little blah, but is it a daily issue for you? It's OK, you can tell me. This is a safe place.

What I am going to ask you to do is to pretend that you love yourself as much as you love your kids. Can you do that? Can you feed yourself as wisely and as lovingly as you'd like to feed your children? If you can do this, you'll be making the next few steps in this process so much easier. The first thing you'll need to do is to ask yourself, what do I know about nutrition? Come on, think back to grade school. What foods make you healthy? Still not ringing a bell? Plants! No not ferns and those weird spider plants that grow like crazy on grandma's porch. How many servings of fruits and vegetables do you personally consume on a daily basis? One, two, six, zero? If the answer is lower than three or four, you have some work to do. It's incredibly simple really. In order to be healthier, you need to eat more plants. In fact, they should be the back bone of your diet. This won't be easy for many of you, but you know it's the truth.

Plant based diets are low in fat and incredibly high in nutrients and fiber. Vegetables are actually the most nutrient dense foods on earth. They are great sources of calcium, iron, vitamin c, magnesium, potassium and even protein. The list of nutritional benefits that we receive from our vegetable friends goes on and on. I'm not going to bore you with it but it is something that has been widely known for a very long time. Side note: by plant based I don't necessarily mean vegetarian. I simply mean a diet that is centered around plants. You choose what kind of proteins you put on your plate. It is a personal choice and no one should judge you for it. As long as the protein is there to keep your muscles strong and able to repair themselves properly. Do you like all vegetables, most vegetables or almost no vegetables? How do you like them prepared? Raw, sautéed, boiled, roasted, baked, grilled or puréed? How many of these options have you tried? Do you feel like veggies are just not your thing and they are a chore to prepare and eat? I'm going to be honest with you here, you're going to have to get over it. Vegetables are a stepping stone to good health. It's how we are built. We need the vitamins, fiber and so on in vegetables to keep our blood flowing smoothly through our veins. They keep us at a healthy weight, keep our vision sharp, give us energy and keep us out of the doctor's office. So, what I want you to do is start with your preferred way of preparing vegetables and try to expand on that little by little. If you love raw salads, try adding one or two new veggies to it along with some new homemade dressings. The internet is boundlessly full of ideas for creating your own crazy delicious salads and very simple dressings. I dare you to go look on Pinterest and not find at least one or two new recipes for your lunch time salad. Do you put meat or nuts in your salad to give it more heft? If not, give it a shot! You'll feel fuller longer and not crave a candy bar or chips late in the afternoon. If you do already add protein to your salads, why not change it up once in a while? Add fish instead of chicken or cashews instead of almonds. If you prefer cooked veggies over raw, start looking for some great new ways of preparing them. Try your hand at kale chips; all the cool kids are doing it. Start experimenting with all the ways you can create the most delicious butternut squash soup recipes to share at holiday potluck get togethers. Really open yourself up to all of the possibilities that the produce section or farmer's market has to offer. This is a time to be brave and adventurous. There are going to be dishes that you don't like or that won't turn out quite the way you hoped but that's kind of the beauty of the art of cooking. Not every creation will be a masterpiece.

It's okay, you're learning. We all deserve to make mistakes when we are learning a new skill or trying something for the first time. But you know what? You are also going to find some amazing new ingredient combinations that blow your taste buds away! You're going to wonder how it is that you've never tried that combination before.

After you've made peace with vegetables, the next step is to add one or two new fruits to your arsenal of healthy choices. Eating fresh or frozen whole fruits everyday are a great way to keep your sweet tooth happy without packing your blood stream with processed white sugar or worse yet, chemical sweeteners that your body has no idea what to do with. So next time you are at the market and going straight for that bag of red delicious apples or navel oranges, take off your blinders. Do a little browsing and pick out just one new fruit that you've never tried before. You don't have to buy a whole bag of something, just one little piece of fruit or a melon that you can share with a family member. It's not a huge investment, but you might just find that you have been missing out on something amazing because you were nervous about trying something new. If you think about it, most foods are going to be new to your kids but you fully expect them to just go ahead and try what you put in front of them. So be brave. Set a good example by showing your kids that trying a new food is not that scary after all. The worse thing that could happen is that you don't like it.

Now I'm going to ask you to do something that is going to make you say, "Huh?". I want you to go back to the store and buy it again. Yep, I said it. I want you to do exactly what we ask of our kids. Try it again. This time sprinkle some cinnamon or a drizzle a bit of honey or peanut butter over it. Do you like it any better this time? If the answer is no, cool. You gave it a shot. If the answer is yes, then you have another go to mid-afternoon snack. Either way, you are showing your kids that you are adventurous, brave and that you don't just try things once and decide you don't like it. Try to do your taste tests in front of them. Make it into a game. Will mom or dad like the fruit? Maybe they can help you come up with ways to try to make the new fruit taste better by suggesting different ingredients to sprinkle over it. See what happened? You just got your kids involved in thinking about trying new foods. Woohoo! Sorry, I get pretty excited about this kind of stuff. Hence the book.

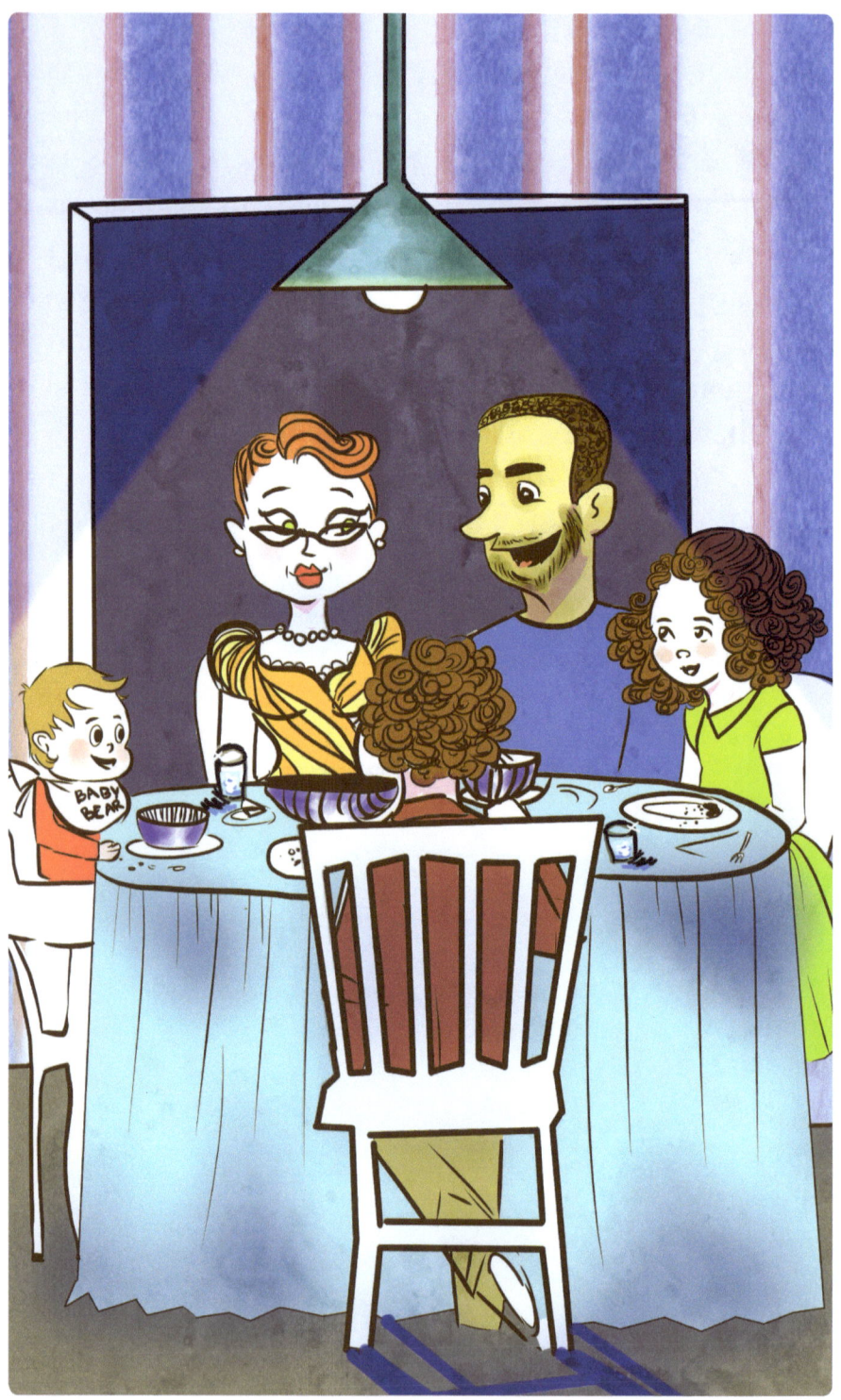

– Chapter 4 –
SERVE, EAT, REPEAT

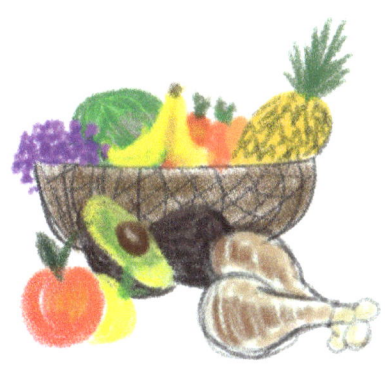

One of the best ways to familiarize anyone with anything is to present it to them over and over again. I know, duh. But really, this is the one sure fire way of getting kids or anyone else to try something they might not otherwise. This is especially true for small children that are just starting on solids. When you put the same dish of sliced avocado or fresh berries on the table at meal time and they see you eating them, they will get curious. That small child will want to try whatever it is that they see mommy and/or daddy enjoying. They'll want to know what must be so good that you are having it every night. It's so important that our kids see us, their idols, eating these nutritious foods over and over again. It programs their little minds to understand that we consider these foods to be just a regular part of our days and our lives.

Along with serving these fresh ingredients daily, we need to talk about their good qualities with our adult partners and our kids. Why are we eating them everyday? What makes them special? Why are we making them an integral part of our lives? It doesn't have to be much, just a few choice words. Carrots are crunchy, sweet and make our eyes see better. Fresh spinach is so green and helps us to be tall and strong. Kids aren't going to understand how each vitamin and mineral effects our bodies and minds. Their eyes will glaze over if we try to make it a lengthy science lesson. They understand taste, texture and how the food will or will not make them grow strong. Of course I'm now talking about pre-school and elementary aged children. Obviously if we are dealing with older kids, we can get a little more in depth with our conversations.

When I say to serve the same things again and again, what I mean is to serve the same couple things as side dishes several days in a row. For example, say it is early spring and asparagus is at its best, put a dish of it on the table each night for a week. You can serve it differently each night. Monday night serve it raw with a dressing for dipping. Tuesday night serve it roasted with butter and herbs. Wednesday have it steamed with a cream sauce. Thursday, try it raw again but with another kind of dipping sauce. All along, you are eating whatever it is that you want for your main dishes. It doesn't have to be boring or monotonous. You are just helping your picky eater to get used to having a new food around and seeing that you really like it. It's also showing them that you can have this strange new food in lots of different and creative ways. Along with the asparagus, you might also put out a dish of fresh fruit. Maybe they've had it already and it's something you know they'll like, or it could be another newbie. Either way, kids are much more likely to try a new kind of fruit than a vegetable. They know fruit is sweet. It's easy; less scary. Again, when you are eating the fruit, talk it up. Is it juicy, sweet, tangy? How does it make you feel when you eat it? Is it refreshing? Does it tickle your tongue? Why not make it a game with the littles? See what words they can use to describe the taste and feel of the foods. For instance my 5-year-old likes to come up with silly words to describe things. This sauce is bloppy, that spice zaps my tongue. Sometimes I have to ask him if his word means it's good or bad but at least he's talking about it.

Ok, so you've put the same two items on the table for a week. Whether your child tried them or not, you now move on to two different foods that you can serve up for a few days. Put them on the table, eat them, talk about them and enjoy them. This process really is as much for you as it is for them. They are being introduced to new healthy foods that they will hopefully one day try and like. You are eating healthy and finding out how you like your fresh foods prepared. This is also a great opportunity for you to eat seasonally. The absolute best time to introduce new foods to your kids is when they are in season in your area. If you live in the northeastern United States, you definitely do not want to give your tot a raw tomato in December. You want their first tastes to be the best they can be. Tomatoes are the freshest and most delicious in late summer. Spring time would be the best time for leafy greens, herbs and plump berries. Peaches and apples are at their absolute best in early fall. This is different for different areas so take the time to get to know your area's growing season. It really does make a huge difference in taste and quality of the produce, to have them locally and in season.

Up until now, you have just been putting the new foods on the table in dishes and taking some for yourself. You have not offered any to your kids. If you are lucky, they have asked to try some or if they are tiny and don't have words yet, they have reached out for them. If they haven't asked for a taste, that's OK. Now you are bringing back one or two of the foods you previously introduced for a second try. This time when you serve up a portion for yourself, put one or two pieces on their plate too. They don't have to eat it but it does have to stay on their plate. They're getting a closer look at it. They can smell it, pick it up, feel it and maybe even lick it. They are getting used to it. No pressure. It's just one or two pieces of something, not a huge waste if they don't actually eat it. Continue with the crunching and talking about how it tastes and feels. By now, they are getting used to how mealtime works. It's about the family enjoying their food together. This should not be torturous for anyone involved. It should be an adventure in discovery. Everyone in the family gets to individually figure out which foods they like prepared in which way. This process is a slow but easy one. There is no pressure on anyone, no anxiety filled meal times. This is just eating and learning. One of the greatest gifts you can give your kids is the love of good food. Teach them how to love and appreciate what food does for them and their health.

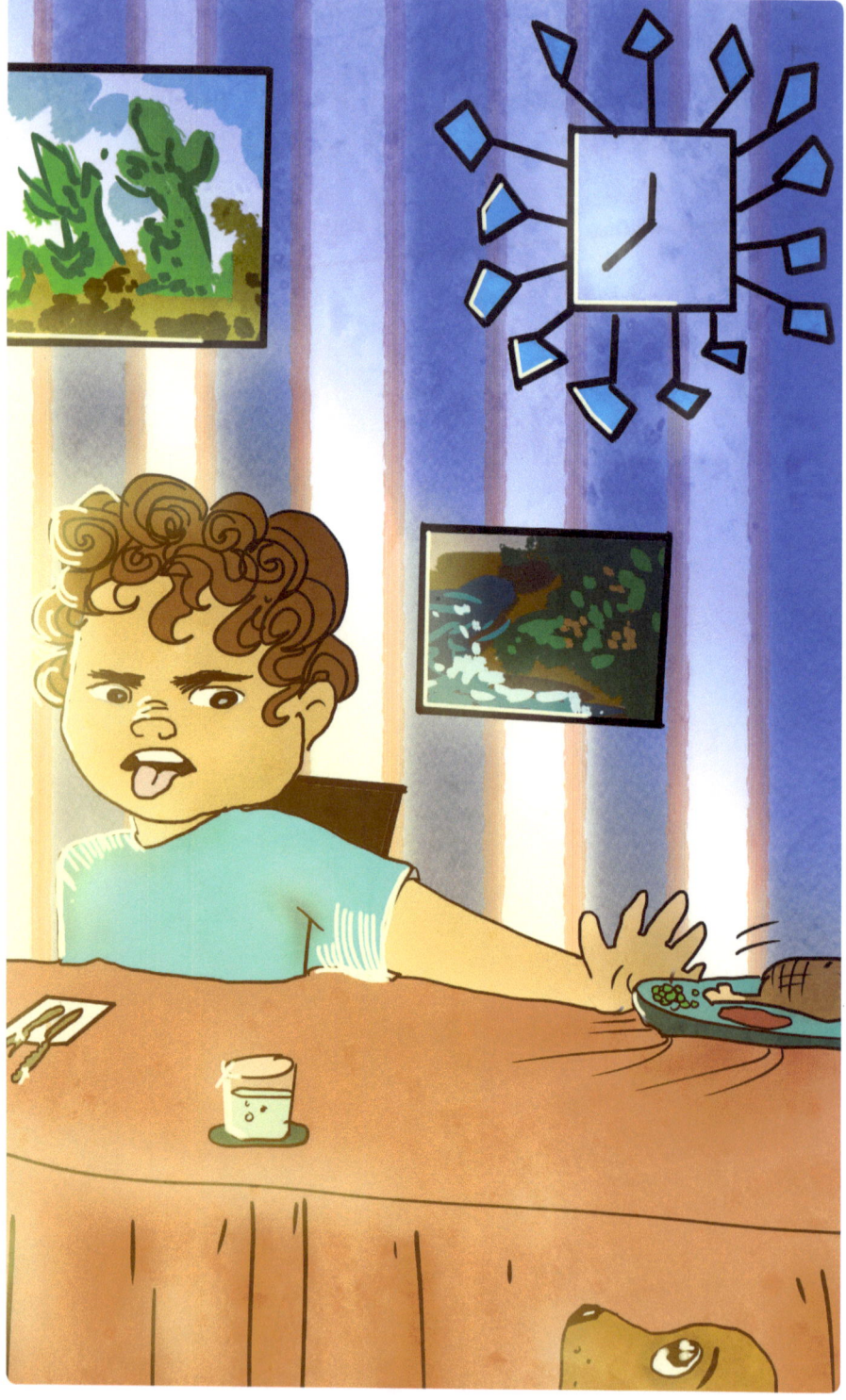

– Chapter 5 –
NO THANK YOU

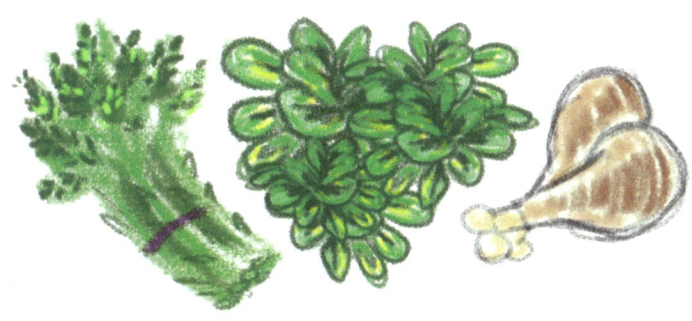

For this next lesson, I want you to ask yourself a serious and very direct question. That question is, "Do I like every food I try?" Be honest now. It's really OK to admit that as an adult, you have tried some foods that just made you want to wretch.

For me, it's okra. I have tried that slimy little veg a few times in my life and I just can't get past the texture. Maybe, I just haven't had it cooked properly or a way that doesn't make my stomach turn. Whatever the case, if I see it listed as an ingredient on a restaurant menu, I avoid it. I know that there must be plenty of lovely people out there who love okra and eat it all the time. I'm just not one of them. Another food that really turns me off is eggplant. Again, I think it's the texture and possibly the innate bitterness that I dislike. I can sometimes stomach eggplant if it is smothered in red sauce and cheese and so much other stuff that I can barely tell that it's in the mix. I do enjoy babaganush because there's no sign of the actual feel or taste of the vegetable left. So there you have it, I've fessed up to a couple of my food don'ts.

What are some of yours? If you can make a list of more than five things, you are 100 percent totally normal.

Why do you expect your kids to like every single thing you put in front of them? It's a bit of a double standard, don't you think?

Yes, there are kids (many, many kids) who turn their noses up to everything that isn't white or made of bread or round. I know these kids. They frustrate parents to no end and make us feel like pulling the hair out of our heads. They make us want to give up on cooking and possibly even parenting all together. These are the kids that have mastered the grand art of Mealtime Manipulation. So much so that if they got their way, they would never touch a fruit or vegetable in their lifetime.

The truth is we all get manipulated by our kids to a certain extent, every day. They're cute, sweet and most importantly, they're ours. Ours to love and care for. We don't want them to suffer, cry or feel that they are lacking something. We want them to feel contentment and happiness as often as possible.

They bank on this. They know they've got us right where they want us almost all the time. They beg, smile, cry, fall down on the floor and beg some more until we either give in or feel like crap for not doing so. I say this with understanding and love. We are not bad parents for falling prey to these adorable little multitalented actors. We are human and very, very tired. We all give in sometimes, just to get some peace and quiet for five minutes. Anyone who says they don't is either a liar or a robot. I haven't met many robots. It's fine that we do that. They need to have a win every once in a while. It gives them hope. However, we are the parents. The ones who keep a roof over their heads (fingers crossed) and that get to make the big decisions for them. Is what they eat on a daily basis a big decision? I think it's one of the biggest. What they are eating now is going to affect who they are as adults. A kid who only eats crackers and pasta is cute, an adult who only eats crackers and pasta is sick and obese.

Kids who refuse to eat anything you would like them to are extremely difficult to deal with at meal time, but not impossible. At our house, when we are putting out a new food, everyone must try it. If they try it and genuinely don't like it, for one reason or another, they don't have to take more. I don't mean one bite of something. I mean a whole green bean or whole slice of cucumber. They need to really taste it. I think we've all sat through the child pretending to take the smallest bird-sized bite of a food they didn't want to try. It's frustrating to say the least. Eating one whole piece of a new food is something that they should get used to doing. It's a way of introducing new flavors, textures and food conversations to the whole family. If they refuse to try it, they lose one privilege that they enjoy that usually happens after the meal. It's very simple. They choose whether not trying the food is worth losing a video game, story time, playing outside or whatever. It's not punishment or torture, although they will disagree. It's us showing how much we care about them. We need to let them know that we are feeding them these great foods because we want them to be strong, healthy, smart and have the best chances possible in life.

The thing to try to remember is that you are not doing them any favors by allowing them to dictate what they will and won't eat. When they are adults buying their own groceries, they can choose what their diet will be. For now, that's your job. You are teaching them and their taste buds to appreciate the freshest, healthiest ingredients and meals that are available to them.

So, you've put out the steamed beets with butter, cinnamon and pecans and they've turned their nose up to it. You tell them that, as usual, they need to eat one whole slice of beet with one pecan piece. If they eat it and decide they didn't like it, you thank them for trying it and they can say, "no thank you" to having anymore that night. That doesn't mean that they never ever have to try another beet at a meal you cook. It means, for that night, they are off the hook. Next time you make beets, they have the same option. One slice of beet, and then they can either finish the serving or say no thanks to the rest. They will either eventually start to like beets cooked in different ways or become very polite about not liking beets at all.

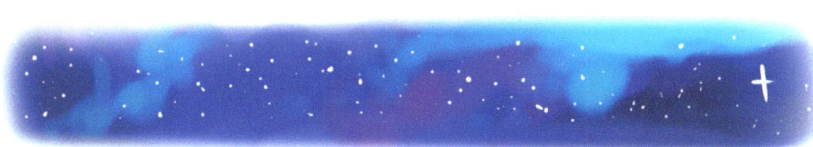

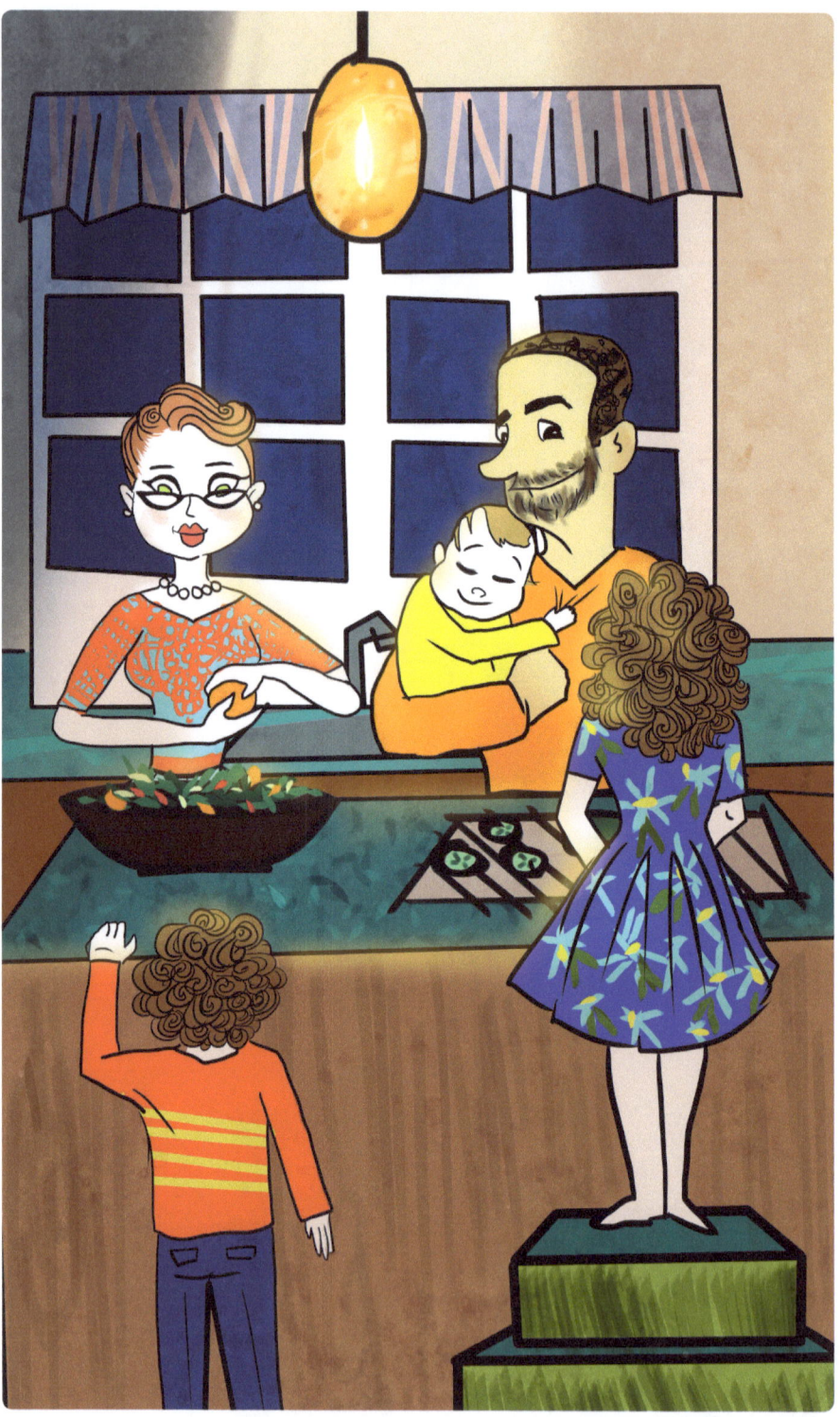

– Chapter 6 –
LITTLE HANDS
IN THE KITCHEN

Scrubbing carrots, rinsing lettuce, washing apples and grapes are things I started doing with my son when he was big enough to reach the sink with the help of a chair to stand on. Eventually we moved on to washing all the vegetables for the weekly salad. Every time he started to wash a new veggie, he would take a bite out of curiosity. He was so excited to be helping and swishing the new colors and shapes around in the cold water, that he just automatically wanted to know what they tasted like. Raw carrots, celery, bell peppers, broccoli, cauliflower and radishes all found their way into his mouth via his own cold, wet hands. It was pretty magical that I didn't even have to coax him to give them a try. He would bite into a whole red bell pepper and teethe on a head of broccoli with no complaints!

He's now five-and-a-half years-old and has graduated to whisking eggs and stirring sauces, but he still loves to come into the kitchen and nab a freshly washed stalk of celery from the sink. Now it's his little brother who stands at the sink with me scrubbing and swishing raw vegetables every week. Before I brought him into the kitchen with me, he didn't "like the green." After helping mama clean the produce, he happily eats lettuce, celery, spinach, kale and green beans! Two out of two kids agree, helping in the kitchen makes food fun. Yep, that's my incredibly scientific study.

This is working on the assumption that you are starting to fill your fridge with fresh vegetables once a week. Even if your kids haven't started eating tons of fresh produce yet, you should be. Having your kids help you open a package of powder mix to add to ground beef doesn't quite have the same effect. You need to get their little hands working with the raw ingredients. New fruits and vegetables that are vibrantly colored and have unique textures really excite kids. That's the element we're looking for here; excitement. Kids want to be entertained and crave things that are new to explore. The best time to open up their world to new, healthy foods is right now.

I'm also working on the assumption that you are willing to take time to spend some special "play" time with your child. If your kids are anything like mine, anytime they get to spend with me is play time. I'd much rather be in the kitchen with them getting messy and passing on my love of food than playing action figure battles again. Sure, there are many elements to working in the kitchen that will remain too dangerous for them to get involved with for several more years, but there are lots of ways for them to help out in meal preparations. To this date, my older son still remembers the time I let him slice up some mushrooms with a butter knife. He felt so grown up because he was actually getting to cut something with a real knife! After that he stopped asking me to cut up his pancakes on Sunday mornings since he already knew how to use a knife. Yay! One less job for me to do at mealtime! When you teach something to a kid under the guise of "fun" they rarely forget it. And when you praise them for how well they do the fun task, they feel pride in what they are doing. They want to feel that pride in themselves and the ability to please you at the same time.

So, set aside some time and get you and your kids working side by side at the sink, cutting board or stove! You will thank yourself for it.

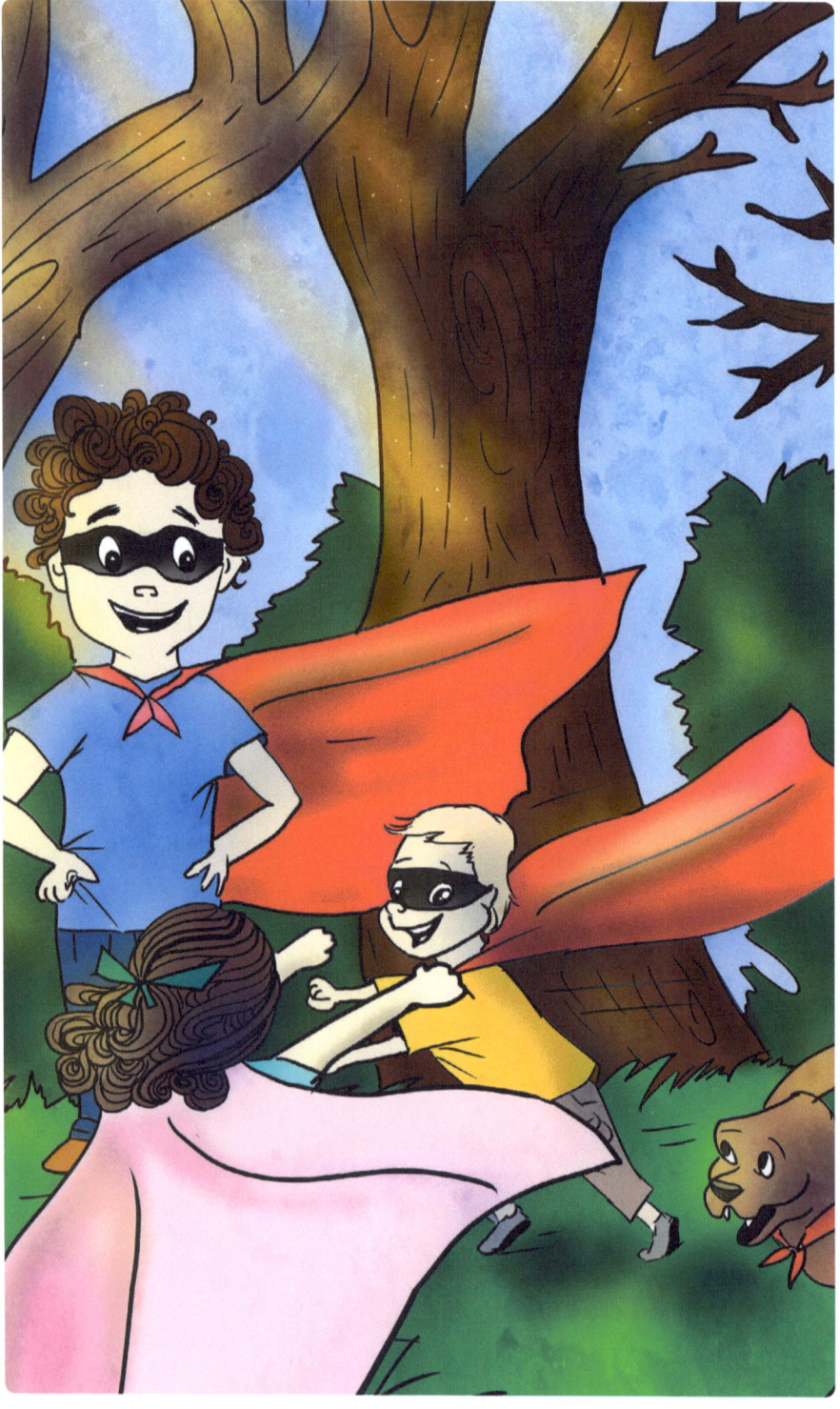

– Chapter 7 –
CREATING TOMORROW'S SUPER HEROES

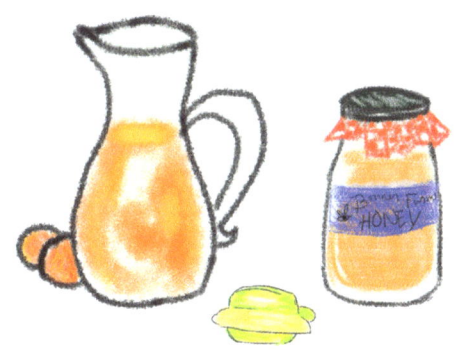

Besides preparing food with my kids, the number one food-positive influence on their little minds has been WWSD. What Would a Superhero Do? I'm serious. The first time my oldest refused to eat peas (his one time arch nemesis) my husband pulled this little gem out of thin air: "You know who loves peas? Darth Vader." My son knew nothing about Darth Vader being a bad guy. He just knew that he was a big cool guy that was really strong and breathed funny. So, if peas were good enough for Darth Vader, they were good enough for him. Even if he only ate four, it worked. This isn't a trick we needed to implement often but it's something that we weren't too proud to use from time to time.

Once he was old enough to understand some more complex concepts (at around three-and-a-half-years-old), we started talking about what foods were highest in vitamins and how they would make him grow faster and stronger if he ate them. He started to learn that the color green had lots and lots of powerful vitamins that helped him to get taller, stronger and avoid sickness. Therefore, when green showed up on his plate, he started to gobble it up first before anything else. At that point, he was really starting to get in to Spider Man, Captain America, The Incredibles and Batman. So naturally we worked those superheroes in to our dinner time conversations. We made the connections between how they must have eaten all of their vitamins in order to get that strong and that fast! He loved the concept of eating the same healthy foods that his idols all ate. He would eat a couple of green beans and say, "Look Mama! I'm getting taller!"

It doesn't have to be superheroes necessarily, it can be anyone your children admire. It could be professional athletes, family members, TV characters or a character out of their favorite book. As long as it is a healthy, strong person that they think is cool.

One little girl told me that she wanted to grow up to look just like her mother and grandmothers. I told her she'd have to eat plenty of fruits and vegetables to be as fast, smart and beautiful as these women. That did the trick for her. She didn't need Wonder Woman for inspiration, just the three most powerful women in her life. She went from eating mostly crunchy, salty white foods to trying more and more fresh new foods everytime I saw her. Now, she loves telling people what her favorite kinds of produce are. I'm super proud of her.

My little guy just turned three and he's still not at the point where we can start teaching about why he should care about vitamins. He's just not there yet and that's OK. Every child is different and learns things at their own speed. He's a lot more work than our first son was as far as food goes. He's very independent and much more strong willed. Apparently, he's a lot like I was as a kid. Yep, my very own mini me (Sorry, Mom and Dad!) But we keep up the positive talk about why we eat the foods we do. It's sinking in there somewhere. I'm not too worried about it. I know that if I'm too tired to keep up the food pep talk for his sake, my big guy will pick up the slack. At five-and-a-half, he's so well versed in nutrients and their value, that it just pours out of him naturally now. When his little brother refuses to try something, he says, "But its so good for you. The protein makes your muscles get bigger and stronger!" or "Eat it, there's so much potassium in those." It can be a little embarrassing sometimes what a little nutrition geek I'm raising. I swear I don't use flash cards! Just daily food conversation.

Like I've said before, to most kids, we are their superheroes. So, we've got to let them know that if they want to grow up to be like Mommy or Daddy, they've got to eat well and exercise often. Again, it's important that we really mean it. Telling them that they need to eat broccoli and carrots to be like us while drinking diet soda and eating a bag of chocolate chip cookies, isn't gonna work. They've got to see it to believe it. So let's show them that we mean what we say! Let's try our darndest to live up to their super standards! Let's really think about what your average (or not so average) superhero is like, shall we? Does Spiderman get drowsy and sluggish when he needs to be out there thwarting bank robbers? Nope. Does Superman get sick from sinus or respiratory infections every other month? Uh uh. Does Black Widow turn down a mission because she's feeling bloaty from digestive issues? Heck no! She kicks butt daily! These are all the health issues that can be avoided through proper nutrition and regular exercise. Issues that a superhero would never have to deal with. Why? Because they eat well, sleep well and move their bodies, Every. Single. Day. At least that's what we're telling our kids.

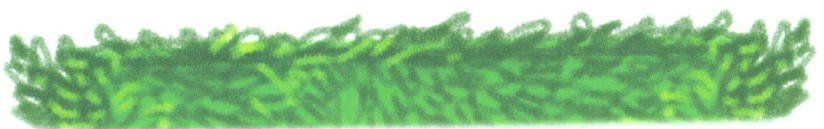

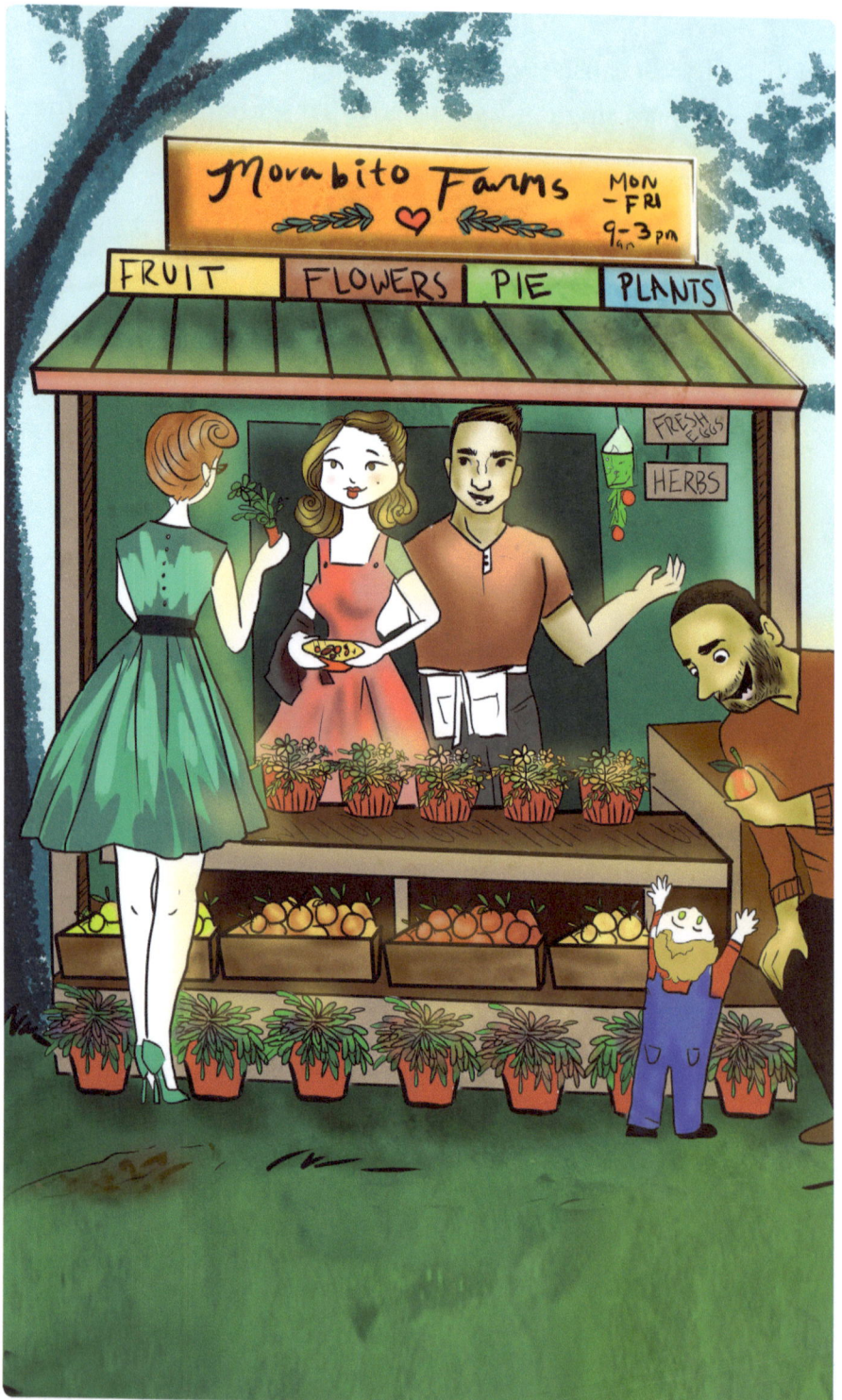

– Chapter 8 –
GIVING THEM THE GIFT OF KNOWLEDGE

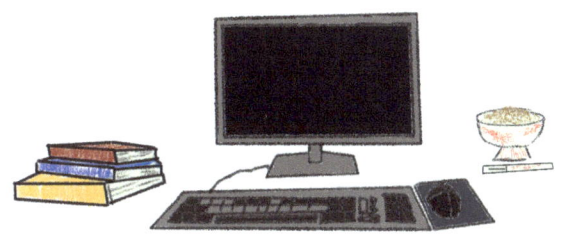

I can't tell you how many times I've had this exact conversation. I'll be out with my kids either at a restaurant or at someone's house and the waitstaff or host will say, "Wow, your kids eat so well!" This statement is always followed by, "You're so lucky, my kids won't eat anything." I smile and say, "Thanks, I guess I am kind of lucky but it was a lot of hard work to get them to this point." I think people really believe that some kids just pop out of their mother's body asking for breast milk with a side of fresh asparagus. If there are parents out there with kids like this, they are truly the luckiest moms and dads in the universe. I am not one of those lucky parents. I made the decision before I even got pregnant with my first son that good nutrition and a healthy attitude towards food was my number one priority as a parent. I decided to learn all I could about what babies, toddlers and kids of all ages need to live healthy lives and to make no compromises in that department no matter what. I pushed myself through the tears and tribulations of breast feeding. I learned how to make fresh baby foods from the very beginning. I made sure that my kids became involved in the process of how I got food to the table. We visited farms so that they could see the animals, fruits and vegetables that we would consume. We met the farmers and picked our own fruits when they were in season. I taught them what the growing seasons in our state are. I taught them why certain foods will make their tummies hurt if they eat too much, why they need to eat more of other things, and why they need to drink water and not so much juice. I explained why I have chosen to become a health coach, teaching other people how to become and stay healthy through nutrition. It's my passion. Ask anyone who knows me, I am a health nut. They'll tell you, it can be annoying.

I'm not asking you to be like me. What I'm asking is that you learn more about health and nutrition and that you pass that information along to your kids. It really is a super thoughtful gift. They might not think so now, but when they are your age, they will be so thankful. I know that they teach health in school but I've got to say I remember next to nothing about what I learned in health class as a kid. I do remember the time the teacher walked around with a section of a black lung in a plastic baggie to keep us from smoking, but that's about it. The things I remember about health from when I was a kid were all the things my mom told me. All the home remedies that she mixed up from ingredients in the kitchen cabinets are still the ones I use today with my own kids. I've known for years how to make my own soup stocks from vegetable scraps and bones from previous meals just by watching her work her magic in the kitchen. Thanks to my mom, I learned about using every bit of our food to reduce waste and get all the nutrients I can out of the basic ingredients. She taught me the miracles of honey and lemon to ease a bad cough. The many, many uses of apple cider vinegar. Did I say many? Trust me, it's amazing.

These are the things I remember from daily life with my mother. These memories have helped me through so many dark days of sick babies and sick me. They were a direct cause of me becoming so interested in nutrition in the first place. I wanted to be as good of a mother and an educator as my mother was for me. What do you remember learning from your parents about staying healthy? What do you want your children to remember about health from daily life with you?

With the internet, magazines and entire TV networks devoted to health and nutrition, the world is brimming with information. Information that is just waiting for you to find it. Now I've got to say that there is a lot of misinformation out there. There are many, many web sites out there that are touting themselves as health experts and sighting non-existent studies to prove their point. Did I say many? You need to keep a clear head and listen to your gut when researching nutrition. If it sounds too good to be true, it is. Every time. If they are selling something, it's a scam. If they are giving you something for free, they want something from you. If they don't give you the information you are looking for unless you buy the "Exclusive Health Program," it's a scam. These are not educators, these are sales people. Go to a bookstore and read some of the books that have interesting titles. If you get a few pages in and it sounds like hooey, it's hooey. If someone is telling you that you need to eat all one way all the time and that their diet will work for everyone, it is a dirty stinking lie!

Everyone's body is different and has different needs. Vegetarian, vegan, paleo, macrobiotic, South Beach, they all work for some people. None of them work for everyone. It's good to explore different dietary theories to know what works best for your body. At the end of the day, you should feel nourished, fulfilled, happy and truly healthy. You should have natural energy that doesn't come from a can, bottle or pill. You should be free of sickness 95 percent of the time. You should have healthy nails, hair and a healthy digestive track on a regular basis. Finally, as a general rule, your meals and snacks should contain fresh, frozen or preserved vegetables and fruits. If you are eating grains, they should be whole (rice, millet, corn, quinoa, barley, oats, etc.) and actually look like a grain. If you are eating meat, it should be free of added hormones, antibiotics and preferably grass fed and local. Nuts, seeds and legumes are awesome if you can digest them. I'm not a fan of drinking dairy but I love butter, cheese and yogurt.

Kids are smart. They absorb everything that they hear and see, whether it's good or bad. You may not think that they will understand a conversation about health and why we should eat certain foods and avoid others but they don't need to. Not at first anyway. They'll see and feel your energy and health getting better. They'll start enjoying spending more time with you in the kitchen. They'll feel the positive shift in your life and the life of your entire family. They'll start asking you questions about the ingredients you use the most and you'll start having answers for them as your research progresses.

All of this can feel overwhelming so just remember these three simple steps for giving your family a healthier lifestyle:

Step 1: Learn what you can about nutrition in the free time that you are willing to dedicate to the topic.

Step 2: As you learn, pass that information on to your children in the most creative, non-threatening way that you can.

Step 3: Feel proud of yourself that you are giving yourself and your kids some incredible knowledge on an incredibly important subject.

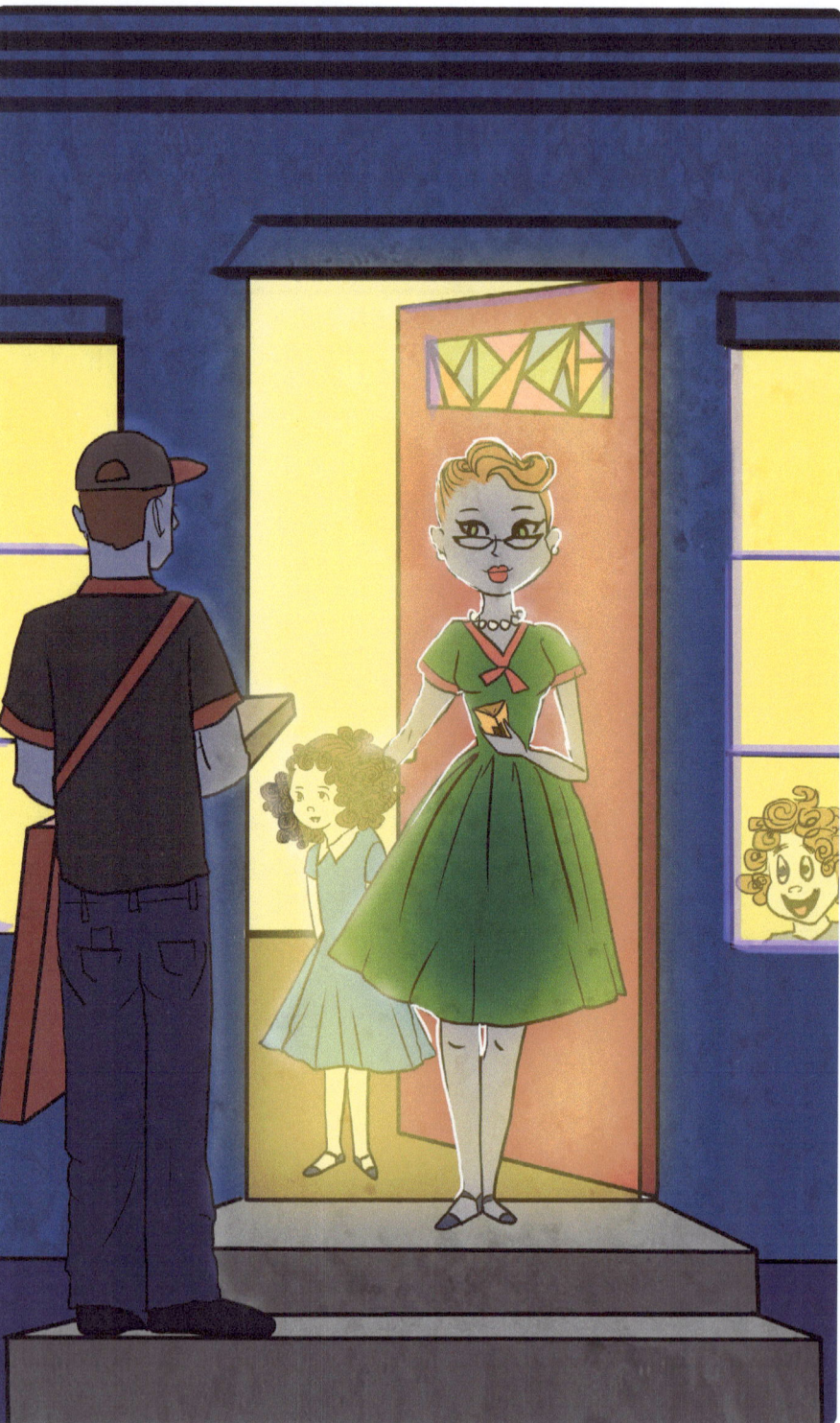

— A Final Thought —
PLEASE REMEMBER, NOBODY'S PERFECT

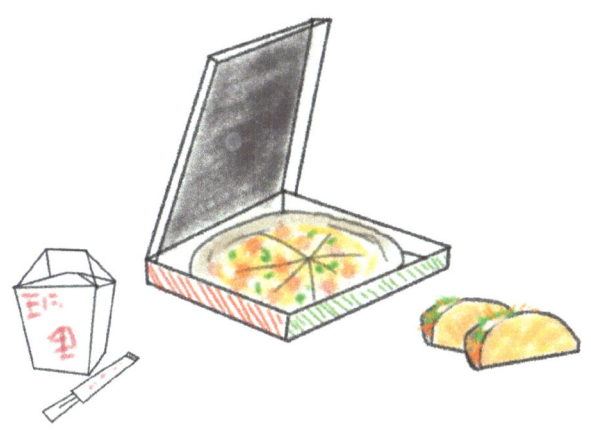

Before moving on to some yummy recipes that you and your kids will enjoy making and eating, remember, this is a process, not an overnight success. Changing the way your family thinks about food has to be gradual if it's going to stick. There will be foods that one or all of your family just can't stomach. There will be nights when there is just no time for a real, fresh meal to find its way to your table because you're on the road between sports practice and a choir concert. There might be times when you are just too exhausted to make one more well thought out meal.

On those nights, give yourself a break. Don't beat yourself up about ordering pizza or stopping at your favorite take out restaurant. Really, it's OK. It's once in a while, not every night. It's allowing yourself to be human and not needing to be a superhero every single day.

My family has a favorite diner, pizza place, Chinese buffet and Mexican restaurant that we go to from time to time. We are not holier than thou, I promise. We are generally very healthy eaters that sometimes indulge in going out to eat. We try our best to make a habit of eating mostly home cooked meals, but like most people, we like a little restaurant food sometimes.

On the occasions that you do get food out, make a real effort to choose the healthier items on the menu if possible. Please don't try to be perfect. It's stressful and isn't realistic. Do your best for you and your kids.

– Recipes –
A FEW FAMILY FAVORITES

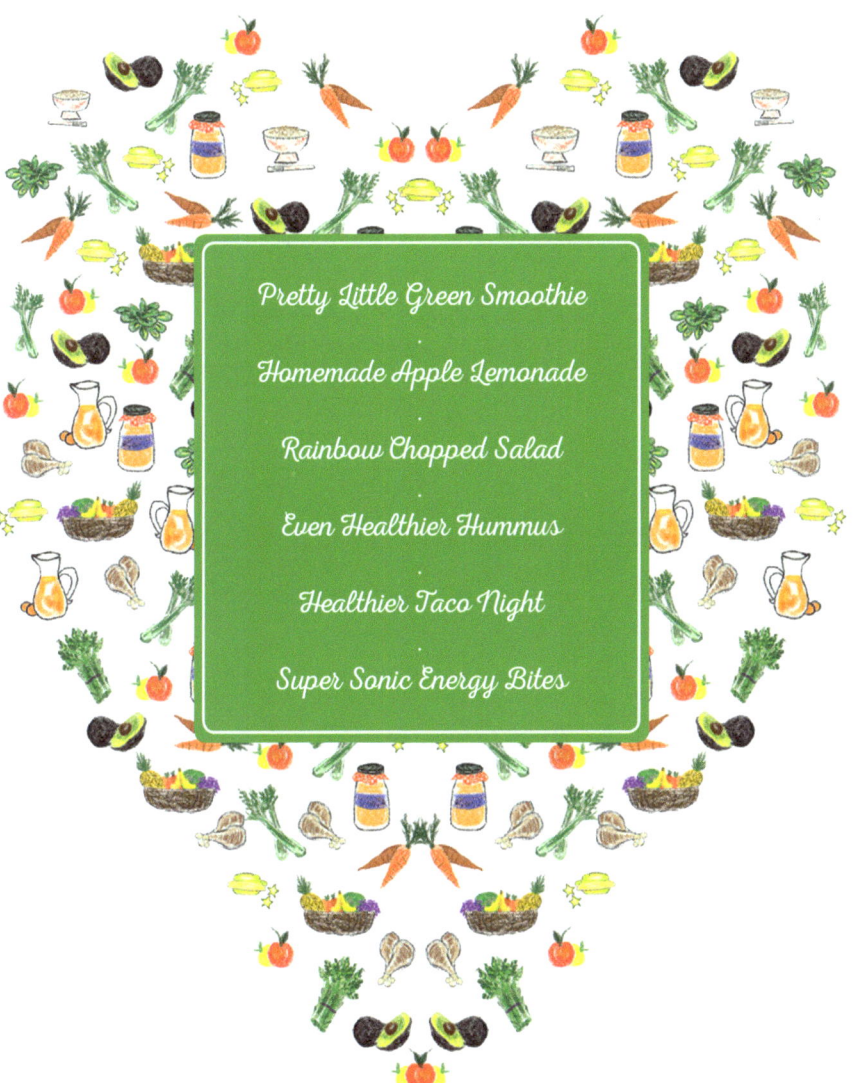

Pretty Little Green Smoothie

·

Homemade Apple Lemonade

·

Rainbow Chopped Salad

·

Even Healthier Hummus

·

Healthier Taco Night

·

Super Sonic Energy Bites

enlightened nourishment.com

Pretty Little Green Smoothie

My kids love smoothies so much, sometimes we have them with dinner. They get their fruits and veggies and a yummy treat all in one! This little gem is simple, sweet and filled with essential vitamins.

INGREDIENTS

- 1 cup original almond milk (any brand)
- 1 cup water
- 1 medium banana
- 2 pitted dates
- 2 handfuls chopped kale
- ½ medium cucumber

DIRECTIONS

Put all ingredients into the blender starting with the wet ingredients first.
Blend on high until smooth and creamy.
Enjoy!

Homemade Apple Lemonade

This is a recipe that I make in the summers when my son starts asking for lemonade. Sometimes I substitute limes for lemons, either way it's not too sweet and very refreshing. The raw honey and lemon boosts the immune system and helps greatly with seasonal allergies. You can add more or less apple juice to your liking.

INGREDIENTS
- 4 average size organic lemons
- ⅓ cup local honey
- 8 ounces organic apple juice
- 1 tall pitcher full of filtered water

DIRECTIONS
Juice lemons and pour juice into the pitcher.
Add apple juice, honey and water.
Stir briskly until honey is fully dissolved.
Serve chilled with ice.

Rainbow Chopped Salad

Salads are great for experimenting. You can add or subtract what you want in order to get all the pretty colors into your kid's bellies. Maybe you can add strawberries instead of dried cranberries. Just remember, the more colors on the plate, the healthier it is.

INGREDIENTS–DRESSING

- ¼ cup apple cider vinegar
- 1½ Tablespoons finely chopped shallot
- ½ Tablespoon honey
- ¼ cup sesame oil
- black pepper to taste

DIRECTIONS

Whisk all ingredients together in small bowl.

INGREDIENTS–SALAD

- 1 big bunch of kale (destemmed and chopped)
- ½ head purple cabbage (sliced)
- 1 large Fuji apple (cored and diced)
- 1 large pear (cored and diced)
- 1 mango (cored and diced)
- ¾ cup sliced almonds
- ½ cup pomegranate seeds or dried cranberries

DIRECTIONS

Combine all ingredients together in large bowl.
Toss together with dressing.

Even Healthier Hummus

Hummus makes a fantastic snack or party dish. t is already full of protein, fiber and iron. This recipe puts it over the top in the nutrient department. It is also another great way to teach your kids that greens can be crazy delicious.

INGREDIENTS

- 1 cup cooked chickpeas
- 1 heaping Tablespoon of tahini paste
- 1 clove garlic
- 2 Tablespoons plain whole milk yogurt
- 2 handfuls of greens
  (spinach, kale...)
- ¼ cup olive or avocado oil
  (or enough so that you get the smoothness that you want)
- 1 teaspoon each of salt, turmeric and cumin
  (or more to taste)

DIRECTIONS

Put all ingredients in blender.
Blend until smooth, adding oil slowly.
Serve with pita chips, blue corn chips or sliced vegetable sticks.

Healthier Taco Night

What are healthy tacos? To me it means using great, fresh ingredients instead of the pre-seasoned packages. I don't really do recipes, I mostly just rely on my sense of smell and knowledge of flavor combinations and start throwing the spices together. It almost always works.

INGREDIENTS

- 1 pound local pasture raised ground beef
- 1 small red onion diced
- 3 cloves garlic sliced
- 4 tablespoons tomato sauce
- ½ cup small broccoli florets
- 1 teaspoon salt
- ½ teaspoon each of black pepper, chili powder, turmeric and cumin (or more to taste)

DIRECTIONS

Brown the beef then add onion and garlic. Sauté until onion is tender.
Add tomato sauce, salt, pepper, turmeric, chili powder and cumin.
Cook for ten more minutes.
Add broccoli florets and cook for five more minutes.

I use the Garden of Eatin' yellow corn taco shells made with organic corn. For toppings I set out medium salsa, plain whole milk yogurt and shredded Mexican blend cheese. Since the taco mixture already had broccoli, I don't feel the need to add shredded lettuce.

Super Sonic Energy Bites

Named by my oldest son after the first time he tasted them, these are the perfect healthy and delicious snack. Fast, easy and packed with power.

INGREDIENTS
- 2 cups pitted dates
- 1 cup raw pumpkin seeds
- ½ cup shredded coconut
- 1 tablespoon cocoa powder
- 1 teaspoon cinnamon
- ½ teaspoon ginger powder

DIRECTIONS
Throw all ingredients into the food processor and blend well.
Scoop out Tablespoon sized portions and roll into balls.
Finally, roll bites in extra coconut, cocoa powder or cinnamon (optional).
Makes approximately 1 dozen bites.

– Recommended Books –
SOME FANTASTIC BOOKS THAT MAKE EATING FUN

A Green, Green Garden
by Mercer Mayer

Eating the Alphabet–
Fruits and Vegetables from A to Z
by Lois Ehlert

The Very Hungry Caterpillar
by Eric Carle

Green Eggs and Ham
by Dr. Seuss

Gregory, the Terrible Eater
by Mitchell Sharmat

The Man Who Cooked For Himself
by Phyllis Krasilovsky

Bread and Jam for Frances
by Russell Hoban

ABOUT THE AUTHOR

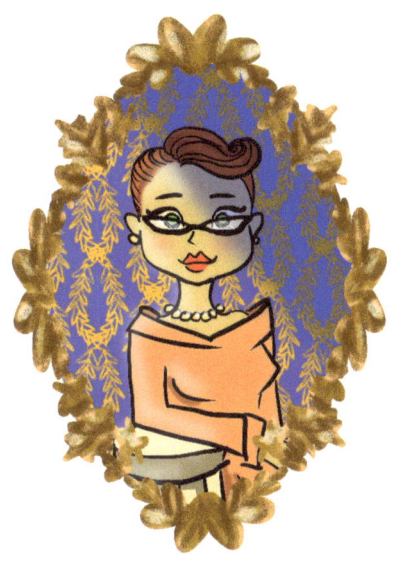

Theresa Bonner is a Certified Health Coach who has received her training and education from the Institute for Integrative Nutrition. She is certified with the American Association of Drugless Practitioners and is a member of the International Association of Health Coaches. Before attending IIN, she was an avid health and nutrition researcher for 20 years. She specializes in educating her clients on how to make the healthiest choices for their individual needs. She guides her clients through setting and attaining the goals that will lead to life changing health and vitality. When she is not working with clients, she is constantly continuing her education in nutrition and coaching techniques. She is also a mother of two young sons who loves to cook, write, eat good food, sing, dance and get involved in her community. She is currently an active board member of the Somerville New Jersey Municipal Alliance and Youth Services Commission.

www.ingramcontent.com/pod-product-compliance
Lightning Source LLC
Chambersburg PA
CBHW040322010626
45792CB00024B/2092